Alcoholics ᴎᴏᴛ Anonymous
A Modern Way to Quit Drinking
By
Paul Trammell

Copyright 2017 Paul Willis Trammell
ISBN 9781521594438

Introduction

Get sober, you'll be amazed at what happens! In the beginning it will be very hard, but it gets easy after a while, and the longer you stay sober, the easier it gets to stay sober, because you will love being sober. Everything in the life of an alcoholic improves when he or she quits drinking. There is nothing to fear, and much to gain. Becoming sober and learning to live a sober life is like recovering from a long illness, like being healthy and happy after years of sickness and depression. It's like emerging from a mud-hole in which you've been mired for years, a mud-hole in which you thought would be fun to play, but instead turned into a devastating trap.

The sober person you are becoming will develop new and wonderful goals, goals which will be achieved. Addiction diminishes our drive to better ourselves, because when we are using, all we want is our drug (or drugs - yes, alcohol is a drug!). But as sober people we experience many enlightenments which cause us to set new priorities that enrich our lives. Sitting around drinking and hanging out in dingy bars is really not very interesting or fun. The world has much more to offer, and sobriety opens new doors, presents new opportunities, and causes us to crave new and interesting experiences.

Sobriety also brings a lot more money. Not only do we realize direct savings from not buying alcohol, but we also realize many indirect financial benefits. No longer hungover every morning, we show up on time for work. Our minds become much more clear and function on a higher level, allowing us to work more effectively and more efficiently. We begin to earn more money. We save more money. We recognize habits that waste money and we eliminate them. We analyze our finances and maximize our earnings. The bottom line is that sobriety pays big.

Alcohol is terrible for our health. It negatively affects all of our organs and crushes our spirit. It kills people. It causes a long slow death in heavy drinkers, and it kills many more quickly - in accidents that would not have happened had the victim been sober. It causes fights. It causes us to make stupid decisions. It makes us eat unhealthy foods at odd times of the night. Cellular changes occur in the bodies of the addicted. The addict no longer wants to eat food, but wants more alcohol all the time. The alcoholic eventually becomes severely malnourished and dies a slow and tragic death. Consider the following:

Over the centuries, alcohol has become the most socially-accepted addictive drug worldwide. Excessive alcohol use is the third leading cause of preventable death in the United States. Although normative alcohol use is ubiquitous, alcohol dependence is a serious medical illness, experienced by ≈14% of alcohol users. Alcohol dependence constitutes a substantial health and economic burden, costing an estimated $184 billion in expenditures stemming from alcohol-related chronic diseases such as heart disease, Alzheimer's disease, stroke, liver disease, cancer, chronic respiratory disease, diabetes mellitus and bone disease, which may develop following chronic alcohol ingestion and contribute to the alcoholism-related high morbidity and mortality. Alcohol abuse may also trigger a cascade of acute health problems such as traffic accident-related injuries, social problem including domestic violence, loss of work-place productivity, economic burden on society, crime and public disorder.

Alcohol use is characterized by central nervous system (CNS) intoxication symptoms, impaired brain activity, poor motor coordination, and behavioral changes, largely as a result of impaired CNS activity due to alcohol's effect on synthesis, release and signaling of neurotransmitters, including serotonin, glutamate, GABA, endocannabinoids and their receptors. Alcohol abuse causes functional impairment of the gastrointestinal tract, liver, and pancreas. It also affects protein, carbohydrate, and fat metabolism, and leads to insufficient immune system responses to infections, impairs the ability of the host to counteract hemorrhagic shock, augments corticosteroid release, and delays wound healing, thus contributing to higher morbidity and mortality, and prolonged recovery from trauma.

from Cellular and Mitochondrial Effects of Alcohol Consumption, Salvador Manzo-Avalos and Alfredo Saavedra-Molina, International Journal of Environmental Research and Public Health, Dec 2010

Alcohol is slavery. Those who make it and sell it are drug dealers. Bars are modern-day opium dens. They know they are pushing an addictive drug and they rely on alcoholics to finance their dark businesses. Sobriety is freedom from this slavery. Getting sober means freedom from craving, and craving is suffering. Happiness will come from sobriety, as will health and wealth. All the pieces of your life that have fallen to the floor will be picked up and reassembled, better than before. You will start growing again. You will improve. Sobriety is the good life, alcoholism is a long slow death.

Please note that while serious alcoholics will require medical attention in order to avoid hazardous and potentially deadly withdrawal effects, this book is about the methods that I used to get sober. This has worked for me and for others, and while I am not a doctor or an addiction professional, I simply want to share my method with the world in the hope that many people will become sober and experience the freedom that I have found.

While the title of this book plays with the name of the world's most successful sobriety-organization, Alcoholics Anonymous, I in no way intend to demean or delegitimize AA. It is an organization that works for many people, and if the methods I lay out don't work for you, then by all means go to AA. You might want to go even if you like my methods, as a reinforcing system.

The Beginning

Relish in your own strength and independence. Our culture accepts an extremely addictive and destructive drug, but we don't have to accept it. Make your own decisions and never do something just because it seems like everyone else is doing it. We must think long and hard about what makes us happy and why these things make us happy. Using this information, we must design our lives accordingly. We do not have to live the lives that society has pushed upon us, for this is what got us addicted to alcohol and has been ruining our lives. The time is now to start to redesign our lives, without alcohol or other drugs.

As you are getting sober, do all the things that alcohol prevented you from doing in the past. Staying sober will create a lot of free time that you may not be used to having. Be productive. Make and save more money. Exercise more, read more, learn something new. Relish in sobriety and reject drinking-society.

There are other sober people around, but at least in the beginning, we tend to be less social. However, if you look, you will find them. This is one reason why I use social media to share my struggle with and disdain for alcohol. I don't want to be anonymous, and helping others quit is part of the therapy.

Stay sober today and build a fabulous and wonderful sober life. Save all that drinking money and go on an awesome adventure with the money you saved. I used the money I saved in my first year of sobriety to take a one-week sailing class, and then I went on a three-week sailing and surfing vacation in the Caribbean. In my second year of sobriety, I bought a sailboat and christened it Sobrius, in order to honor my sobriety, and to constantly remind myself of my commitment to stay sober. As I write these lines, I am sitting at the navigation table of Sobrius, drinking fruit juice and enjoying some of the best times of my life, and some of the best health of my life.

We have to force ourselves, in the beginning of our sober life, to do the things that we want to continue doing but that we needed alcohol to help us do in the past. If the activity is something we legitimately enjoy, then it will come, if it was foolish then you will know it and let it go. I used alcohol and marijuana to help me perform onstage. I am a musician, a guitar player in a band, and I drank and smoked whenever I played. I was afraid that I might not enjoy playing music as a sober person, but I adapted.

Performing sober was tough at first, although it became easier with time and experience. Playing music is legitimate, fun, and rewarding, so I still enjoy it without alcohol or marijuana. However, staying out late at bars and talking to drunk people is not so legitimate and only fun if you too are drunk, therefore I don't do this anymore. Change is good.

Think about the things you used to do only when drinking. Ask yourself if you gained from them. Some will be positive and beneficial, and you should keep doing these things, even if it takes a new effort to do so. Other activities you may determine were only excuses to drink, or were only done as a result of being drunk and were destructive. You don't need to do these things anymore. This is your new life and you must design it well.

We live in a strange world containing many obstacles to overcome and rise above. As a sober person, you will have an edge on all the drinkers, and you will gain super-powers. You will conquer all obstacles and achieve any goal you set, but remember to set goals that will result in personal fulfillment.

Do whatever it takes to stay sober. It is THE most important thing in your life right now. The alcoholic part of your mind might try to trick you into thinking that some important thing in your life requires alcohol to do or achieve. But this is not true. You can do and achieve anything without alcohol. If something in your life is threatening your sobriety, step away from it. Perhaps you will go back to this activity or event in the future when your resolve to stay sober is stronger, but in the beginning, just step away. Nothing should get in the way of your getting and staying sober. The rest of your life depends on this. Make staying sober your number-one priority.

Don't expect others, especially non-addicts, to understand our struggle. I often say to them, when they tell me they don't have a drinking problem, "I wish I was like that, but I'm not. I can't just have a couple of beers. You're lucky to be able to control your drinking." Those that are not prone to addiction and don't have experience with recovering addicts don't understand our position. To them, drinking responsibly comes naturally. They don't have the devil on their shoulder telling them to drink all day long. They might go through an entire week without thinking about drinking. This is not the life we live, and ours is not the life they live. So don't expect them to understand what we are going through, don't judge them for their ignorance, and don't take their ill-founded advice. Rather, be ready for them by thinking ahead. Anticipate that someone someday will tell you that you can drink responsibly, and be ready to explain to them why you can't.

Also, remember that you are not obligated to go to social events. Alcoholism is very serious and staying home is perfectly acceptable. When in doubt, don't go out.

Cravings

Cravings will occur frequently in the beginning. Remember that alcoholism is a disease, or a condition, both mental and physical. These cravings are a symptom of this disease, and you must recognize this. Cravings are not a weakness of yourself, nor are they a true desire. They are simply a symptom of your disease. You can overcome cravings with mental effort. Tell yourself that you are stronger than the craving and that you will defeat it. In a short time, it will pass, and you will have scored a victory.

Each time you overcome a craving, recognize it as a success. Each time you succeed, your disease grows weaker, but you must recognize the victory and congratulate yourself for it. Do this consciously.

Redirect your attention and energy to something productive, like exercise. Exercise is a good substitute for drinking, as it is a positive activity that can satisfy some of the same needs that you were using alcohol to satisfy in the past.

Realize that these cravings have no value. They are not something you need to follow. They are like the devil's advice. Do the opposite of what these cravings demand.

Cravings come on hard and fast. They must be anticipated and planned for. First, always know that they will pass. Cravings have a way of making you think that they will go on forever, leading us to feel like we are going to have to resist them all day. This is not true; the craving will pass as quickly as it came on. You simply must resist and wait it out. You will find that as soon as you start resisting, a strength grows inside you. Every second you resist the craving is a success, and your confidence will build as you resist. As your confidence and strength are building, the craving is diminishing. You are winning, and the craving is losing. The craving passes and you get on with your life, stronger and more confident for the struggle.

Relapse

If you relapse, you must learn from your mistakes and keep going. All of your progress is not lost. Just figure out how it happened and make a new strategy to prevent it from happening again. You can do this; you don't drink anymore. You have not lost the battle.

A relapse should also make you consider adding to your strategy. It could be that you need professional help, or perhaps you should attend an Alcoholics Anonymous meeting. Whatever the case, you need to reevaluate your strategy and do whatever it takes to get sober. Think critically about why you relapsed and figure out how to get through the future without it happening again.

Challenging Situations

What doesn't make you drink makes you stronger. Of course, some days are very challenging. When faced with a particularly hard situation in which to stay sober, consider it a challenge. Realize that staying sober in the future will be easier once you successfully get through this challenge. It will make you stronger and future situations easier. Tell yourself "If I can get through this, then I can get through anything." The more you stay sober, the stronger you get, and the easier it gets to stay sober.

I remember one gig in particular that was very difficult for me. It was the first show my band played after I had quit smoking pot. I had already been sober for a year, but I had only recently quit smoking. I was so used to being high when I played the guitar and performed onstage that I was very anxious about this gig. We would always get high backstage, even though it was an outdoor gig at a marina and we might be seen. We'd sneak a toke behind the stage or go to one of our cars and smoke out in the parking lot. It was really part of the gig experience for me, and fit in nicely with our reggae music.

The challenge was immense; I wanted to smoke but I did not. Before the show, when I would normally be getting high, I walked around the marina and looked at sailboats, which represented a future reward for staying sober. I also called my father, which strengthened my resolve, since he represents strength of character. These activities were substitutes and I used them as tools to battle my craving.

I considered it a challenge and I could tell that if I got through the gig without smoking then I would be able to abstain throughout the future, because nothing was likely to be harder than this. I was right. If you can get through the hard times, all the other times are easy.

The Devils

Feed the devil and it will grow, starve the devil and it will go.

A little devil used to sit on my shoulder, chirping in my ear all day. It would say "Wouldn't a beer be nice now?" Or "You don't have enough beer in the fridge to get you through the night. You better stop at the liquor store and pick up a 12-pack." Around noon every day it would say "What time is it? Is it late enough in the day to have a beer? It's past noon, so go ahead." Late at night it would say "Get another beer, don't be a wimp!" It would tell me things like "You can do whatever the hell you want to do, so drink up. No one can tell you what to do!" - how ironic that it was telling me what to do all along.

I had another devil on my other shoulder who would whisper seductively to me things like "How about a bong-hit?" or "You ought to bring some weed with you to work today." When my bag was getting low it would say "You are almost out of weed, you should get more now. Don't run out!"

These two devils harassed me all day every day. I couldn't control them at all, they just talked and talked, and I had no choice but to listen, or so I thought. They slowly grew stronger every time I gave in to them, which was all day every day. However, they are both gone now. I quit giving in to these little devils, and they grew weak, and then they died. Good riddance!

But at first, they were strong and they put up a good fight when I was getting sober. They yelled at me "You little punk! Get a beer!" "Smoke some weed now!" But I didn't give in to their rude demands, I ignored them! Eventually their voices grew weaker and now they are gone completely. I had power over them all along, I just had to decide to use it.

I had accepted a hard-partying lifestyle as an identity. Defying the devils threatened that identity, and thus threatened me. When we have to change, we have to change our attitude first. I had to decide that I didn't have to be a hard drinking and pot-smoking person, and that I didn't want to be this person anymore. I had to create a new identity for myself, and drawing on past strengths within me, I did just this. My new identity was to be healthy, smart, responsible, and high-achieving. But I needed something exciting too, to replace the excitement of heavy drinking and smoking. So, I decided to step up the outdoor adventure in my life. This fit with the strategy of doing things that I could not do before I got sober, like backpacking, long canoe trips, and sailing offshore.

Why I Continued to Drink for So Long

I used to tell myself that I didn't like the sober version of myself. I remembered sobriety as causing me to be serious and boring, never smiling or laughing, and certainly not making anyone else laugh. But after two years of sobriety I find myself happy, smiling, laughing, overcoming obstacles, not losing my temper, and getting through each day without having to face all the hassles that a life of heavy drinking brings. I think it must be common for addicts to believe that their drug of choice makes them better people and enhances their lives. It has become our friend, after all. We wouldn't want to abandon our good friend, now would we? It is not our friend. It is the enemy - a wolf in sheep's clothing, a devil masquerading as an angel.

Indeed, our good friend, the drug, reminds us daily of how bad things will be without it, and it reminds us that it can instantly cure most any ailment. Anxiety creeps up, our drug stops it in its tracks. Depression looms, our drug takes the edge off. Depression gets worse, alcohol makes us gloriously unconscious. We wake up hungover, another drug takes the edge off in a vicious cycle that feeds on itself like a snake consuming its own tail.

I used to wake up hungover every day and I smoked pot to cure the nausea. I would kick myself for drinking so much and ask myself why an evening of drunkenness was worth the price of being nauseous for most of the next day. The math simply didn't work. Then by noon I would be asking myself if it was late enough in the day to have my first beer. The devil that is addiction berated me continuously, giving me no rest until I had an open beer in my hand and enough in the fridge to get me through the night.

There is no logic that can explain this cycle, because the drug is controlling it.

Sobriety is freedom from the devil, freedom from self-delusion, freedom from sickness, nausea, and hangovers. Sobriety gives us the power to think for ourselves and create a new life. Sobriety gives us health to live our new lives well. Sobriety is the key to a new and better life.

I was also afraid that if I quit drinking I would cease to enjoy some of the things that I lived for, specifically playing guitar in my band. We performed mostly at bars, surrounded by drunks and drinking heavily ourselves. I always drank when I played guitar, whether I was performing on stage or practicing by myself. I loved and looked forward to practice-night with the band. We always drank and smoked weed at practice. We laughed and jammed and had a great time, living the rock-star dream, and doing what the rock-star image in our heads told us to do.

Touring with the band was a non-stop party. We all went into "tour mode" and drank ourselves into oblivion, even to the detriment of our performances. Of course I was scared that if I quit drinking I would no longer enjoy touring.

The band has indeed required a difficult transition for both me and my band members, who thankfully have been supportive. Playing sober was very difficult and scary at first. But I told myself that if this was something that I really loved, then I would love it without the drugs. And I do love it still. I just had to learn to perform and practice sober. Now I play better than ever. Alcohol reduces dexterity, which guitar players need in abundance. Alcohol also reduces one's mathematical ability, and music is math. This was but another challenge in my life that caused me to grow. Sobriety brings growth. We stop growing mentally when we become dependent on a drug, and we pick up where we left off when we get sober.

Why I Quit

I always knew I had a drinking problem, and I wanted to quit for at least a couple of years before I finally did. Alcohol caused a lot of problems throughout my otherwise idyllic life: arrested for a fake ID at 17, a DUI at 19, a stint of getting out of bed while unconscious and peeing in the wrong places (while thinking I was in the bathroom) during college, various failed relationships, thousands of dollars wasted, thousands of hangovers, poor grades in school, an expanding belly, broken bones, missed opportunities, illnesses I would have otherwise beaten…

I tried quitting in high school, before it really got out of hand. But this did not last long at all - I was talked out of it by a friend. This same friend convinced me to drink and smoke weed after I'd been sober for two years in college. Friends like this must be avoided. Sobriety, for an addict, is much more valuable than a friendship with someone who would do this. But I must say that he and I are still friends and I am trying to get him to quit drinking now!

It was eventually a combination of events and circumstances that finally got me to give sobriety another try.

I was at a party at my neighbor's house, the annual Superbowl-Sunday party, with a beer in my hand when I saw my friend Jim. I smiled big and said "Hi Jim! Wanna beer?" as his hands were empty.

As we shook hands he said "No thank you, I've been sober for over a year now."

"Wow!" I said "That's awesome! How'd you do it?" I was always awed by those that had conquered the drink, and curious about how they did it.

"Well" Jim replied, a serious countenance replaced the smile on his face as he looked me in the eye "It started because my brother drank himself to death last year."

His brother was younger than me. I was 44 at the time. Jim's brother didn't die from one episode of drinking too much, rather he died slowly from a lifetime of heavy drinking. Towards the end, he must have known that he was killing himself, and he must have been powerless over the alcohol.

The next day I skipped work, as I was suffering from a horrible hangover. I barely left my room all day. Instead I sat and watched Netflix, surfed the web, and even ordered a pizza, which I never do. The pizza was horrible. It didn't even seem like real food, and it made me sick(er).

I had previously been thinking about using a counselor to quit drinking, and I knew my health insurance would cover it, so I picked up the phone and called a therapist that I knew. I had seen her in the past for something unrelated, but that's a different story.

It turned out that she had a cancellation and I could see her that very day. However, she told me that she was not a substance abuse counselor. I didn't care. She was good-looking and I just needed someone whom I trusted to make my decision seem real - someone to be accountable to, to share my success with, should I have any success to share.

I also asked my brother to check up on me. He said he'd do anything he could to help, so I asked him to call or text me regularly and ask me if I was still sober. This is an extremely helpful strategy. Being accountable to someone else takes the pressure off of yourself. If you try to get sober completely by yourself, you may eventually feel like nobody cares and that nobody will notice if you start drinking again. This is also the person with whom you will share your daily success. When they ask if you are still sober, you will respond with "Yes! I am, and thanks for asking!" because you will be so happy to have someone that cares to ask.

Getting sober is a daily struggle, sometimes more. Each day you stay sober is a HUGE SUCCESS! Someone else needs to acknowledge this.

Having someone checking up on you also reminds you daily that if you relapse then there will be this person who will ask and hope you are still sober, this person taking time and expending energy to help you get sober that you don't want to let down. You want to be able to say "Yes!" and hear them say "That's great, congratulations! Keep up the good work."

Find someone to do this for you. Someone in your family that you love and respect is ideal. Otherwise try to find someone who has gotten sober and is willing to help. Use social media, ask if one of your friends is in recovery and will send you a daily message like "still sober?"

The Not Anonymous Method

- Make a conscious decision to give sobriety a chance.
- Don't drink today, or if this seems to hard, just don't drink right now… or right now… or right now…
- Pour any alcohol that you have in the house into the toilet and take a picture or video of this.
- Use substitutes, like seltzer, fruit juice, cookies, adventure, and exercise.
- Keep count of your days, months, or years sober.
- Get counseling if necessary (your health insurance might cover it).
- Tell someone you are doing this and ask them to check up on you daily.
- After about a week, tell everyone, come out on social media, like Facebook, and let the world know; use it for support.
- Be open, frank and honest when talking to others about your sobriety, don't hide it.
- Do things that alcohol prevented you from doing.
- Use the money you saved by not drinking for a reward, like a vacation.
- Help others get sober.
- Celebrate every month on your sober anniversary, and celebrate big on your yearly anniversary.
- Don't go back to drinking, ever. It's all or nothing. Remember this.
- Don't preach to others who drink, just lead by example.
- Make your dreams come true, and remind yourself that sobriety led you to your dreams.
- Tell yourself "I don't drink anymore".

Make a Conscious Decision to Give Sobriety a Try

If you have a drinking problem, then you know it. You've known it for some time and have probably thought about quitting, but you don't know how to go about doing it. Perhaps you feel like sobriety is impossible, an unattainable goal. Perhaps you've deluded yourself into thinking that you were meant to be a drinker, or that you wouldn't enjoy life or like yourself as a sober person. Let me assure you that this is not the case.

Alcohol is a very insidious drug and its addictive nature takes root in our mind and body and continues to mislead us, making us believe that we should keep drinking forever. When we realize what is happening here and begin to think objectively about it, then we become able to start to make a firm decision to give sobriety a try. Ask yourself the question "why do I drink?" and come up with honest answers. You'll likely be surprised by your responses, and one of them is probably "because everyone else does", which is never a good reason to do anything.

Most of us use alcohol because it's a shortcut to having a good time. It doesn't take much mental effort to have fun while drinking, it just requires the drink and maybe a friend. But there is no growth from this, it's just a mindless activity that's fun in the present and bad in the future. More fun can be had from activities arising from sober thought and planning, and the hangovers are avoided. Sobriety opens doors and brings good health, both mental and physical. Sobriety helps us avoid pitfalls, like car accidents, DUI's, overeating, bad decisions, depression, fights, obesity, poverty, anxiety, accidental death, and countless health problems etc. Not only does sobriety allow us to have much better experiences, it also allows us to fully remember them, and in the end, memories are all we have.

Alcohol is an addictive drug. We are constantly misled by media, entertainment and advertising that alcohol is fun, safe, and an integral part of our culture. For example, you'll often see or hear the phrase "drugs and alcohol" as if alcohol is not a drug. It is a drug. It is the most destructive drug known to man. Yet the media continues to push it on us, whether for the profit of the alcohol industry or for the profit of the media source. The result of this exposure is that we become brainwashed into thinking that alcohol is a rite of passage and a necessary means of attaining adulthood, glamour, femininity or masculinity. It becomes attached to things like sporting-event attendance, the end of a work-day, weddings, holidays, friendship, success, weekends, and the list can go on forever. The important fact here is that we must recognize this and decide for ourselves what we want to do. Letting media control our minds is both unwise and unhealthy. Removing the influence of advertising and product placement is a sound strategy in the effort to quit drinking. Advertisements come in many forms and are created by professionals who know how to get into our heads and create needs within us. Advertisements don't necessarily inform us, rather they create a market for a product. They create a desire within us for things we don't need. Therefore it is helpful to not watch television, movies, or listen to commercial radio while going through the early phase of giving up alcohol.

Don't Drink Right Now, or Right Now, or Right Now...

Great achievements come from baby steps. At some point, someone placed a brick on the ground, and thus began the construction of the Great Wall of China. Likewise, your journey to sobriety will start by simply not drinking today. If this seems too difficult a task, then simply don't drink right now. If you are able to not drink right now, then consider this a success. You have just won a significant battle with your adversary - addiction. Your addiction is now weaker and you are now stronger - congratulations! Whenever you feel the urge to drink, do this again - don't drink right now, and recognize your victory.

Do not think about not drinking tomorrow until tomorrow. Don't ponder future situations in which you would normally drink. The devil that is addiction will use future events to fool you into thinking that it is hopeless to remain sober at these events. Therefore, the devil says, "why go through the discomfort of not drinking today when you are going to have to drink at this future event anyway?". The devil wants you to think that staying sober is hopeless; the devil is a liar.

But the devil is a good liar and can be quite persuasive once you start listening to him. Don't listen. Recognize that the part of your brain that has become dependent on alcohol (or whatever drug you may be addicted to) is trying to convince you to give in. Don't give in, resist. Don't drink right now and don't think about the future, just be here now, be sober now, be victorious now!

It may happen (hopefully not!) that someone will tell you that you are not an alcoholic, that you don't need to quit. Do not listen to these people! They are likely trying to justify their own addiction by denying yours. You must distance yourself from them, at least for now. If you can't avoid them, or must talk to them, you can disarm them by saying something like "Alcohol has caused a lot of problems for me" or "It's best if I don't drink". These are phrases that are hard to contradict, as opposed to saying "I'm an alcoholic and therefore I can't drink" to which they might respond "You're not an alcoholic". Sometimes people will tell us that they only drink two beers a day, or some such reasonable amount, to which I may reply "I wish I was like that, but I'm not. For me, it's all or nothing."

Alcoholics Anonymous espouses the phrase "one day at a time". This is to remind us not to drink today, or as I say "don't drink right now... or right now...". The point is not to think about the hurdles of not drinking in the future. It is common for us to become overwhelmed with thoughts about future events where we will surely face difficulty or awkwardness by not drinking. Don't even start thinking about these things. This is the demon inside you that is alcoholism trying to convince you to give up. Cross those bridges when you come to them, and cross them you will! But for now, not drinking today is the only goal. And if not drinking today seems too hard, just don't drink right now, or right now, or right now...

If you know you must go to some event in the near future where people will be drinking, a bit of planning is in need. Anticipate difficult situations and have solutions ready. If you need to go to a party during the holidays, a family gathering perhaps, which can't be avoided, have an escape plan and key phrases ready to go.

What are you going to say if someone offers you a drink? Think about this ahead of time and have a response ready. Come up with something to say that you are comfortable with. You might want to be straight-forward and smile and say "No thanks, I quit drinking!" or you might feel more comfortable being vague and leaving it at "No thanks". If you are going to be driving, this is always a good reason to give for not drinking. Trying to lose weight is another reason to give if you don't want to come out about it yet. But remember, being open and frank about quitting drinking has two big benefits. The first is that it gives others who care about you the opportunity to support you. The second is that it gives other alcoholics and problem drinkers hope that they too can quit; you are giving them an example to follow.

Anticipate that at some point someone will try to tell you that it's okay to have just one or two drinks. They might reason that since you've been sober for a while that you have demonstrated great willpower and therefore can handle responsible drinking. When people say things like this, they are either demonstrating their own ignorance or they are supporting their own denial of their drinking problem. They might be trying to justify their habit and your sobriety might threaten their justification. The demon inside them is making them try to convince you to drink.

Some alcoholics are made to feel uncomfortable around those of us who have quit drinking, as our sobriety is forcing them to confront their own alcoholism. They'd rather believe that everyone drinks. Remember that our openness to being sober helps them by showing them that sobriety can be achieved; alcohol can be overcome. Even though they may be fighting us on the outside, we are helping them on the inside. When others are drinking around us, it's helpful for both us and them if we have a non-alcoholic drink in our hand. This puts them at ease and makes us feel less like an outsider, and they will remember the non-alcoholic drink you were enjoying. It will serve as a reminder that they too can quit drinking.

Anticipate difficult situations and conversations and have phrases and escape plans ready to go. If I need to, I remind people that I'm different from them. I say to them "I can't control my drinking like you, I wish I could, but I simply can't", and the sideways compliment disarms them. I often say "I wish I could just have a few beers and be responsible, but I can't. If I had one today, I'd be waking up the devil inside me and by next week I'd be back to drinking twelve a day."

Another useful phrase is "Alcohol has caused a lot of problems for me. I'm done with it." You can always fall back on "I'm not drinking today" or "I'm not drinking right now."

If people try to belittle your problem, go ahead and tell them how much you used to drink. Don't be scared; they need to know the extent of your alcoholism if they think it wasn't a big deal. I go right ahead and say "I used to drink 8-12 beers every day. I never went a day without drinking this much, and I woke up hungover every day. I'd smoke pot in the morning to take the edge off the hangover, and by noon I wanted a beer. I was always intoxicated, and sick half the time. I don't ever want to go back to that life, and trying to drink one beer now would put me right back there tomorrow." If people persist in trying to convince you to have a drink, it's perfectly acceptable to go ahead and punish them with a verbal assault and walk away from them, for good. You don't need that in your life and they need to know that such behavior is unacceptable.

Another good strategy is to show up early to a party. Be there to make your rounds and socialize before everyone gets drunk. Enjoy time with your friends, family, or co-workers while they are still reasonably sober, and leave before they all get drunk. As you experience life as a sober person, you will come to realize how ridiculous drunk people look and behave.

When attending social events, have escape plans. If you can, drive by yourself to the event so you can leave whenever you need to. If you need to leave right away, do it. Staying sober is way more important than saying goodbye to everyone. Know how you are going to leave and how you are going to get home and do it before things get ugly. If cravings come on, you might need to leave right away. If you start thinking about having a drink, this will be a red-flag signifying that it is now time to execute the escape plan. If you want a drink, stop and think. Think about your escape plan and then leave.

Also have small escape plans ready, for escaping from

conversations which are getting uncomfortable. If someone is trying to convince you to drink, have a plan ready so you can walk away. A fake phone call might do the trick. Pretend to notice an appetizer that you really want and go get it. You can look over the offender's shoulder and pretend to see someone that you need to talk to, wave to the fake person, say "Excuse me, I need to talk to this person" and walk away. And if it comes down to it, chastise the person for suggesting you drink. Let them know that this is unacceptable and you will not stand for it. Maybe your response will prevent them from doing this in the future and help you or someone else.

Pour it Down the Toilet

If you have any alcohol in the house, and you are feeling strong, pour it down the toilet -where it belongs. Immortalize this moment with a photo or video. Watch this scene intently, and record it in your long-term memory. Think of the money you spent on this alcohol as it pours out. This is a small investment you are now making in your future. This is the best money you ever invested, because sobriety pays BIG! In the future when you feel a craving to drink, remember this scene of the beer, wine or liquor (cocaine, pills, heroin...) pouring into the toilet like the excrement it is; no longer something to be ingested, this foul substance is only suitable only for the toilet.

When you are finished, flush the toilet and watch it go down the drain. Imagine that your addiction is following, because part of it is going down the toilet with the alcohol.

Wash your hands. You don't drink anymore.

If you took a photo or video of the pouring out of the alcohol, post it on social media and tell your world that you are quitting drinking. You will get support from your friends and from any of your acquaintances who have also quit. You are one of them now. Use this for support. Share your trials and tribulations; share your successes too. Recognize those who give and offer support as your true friends - your new team that will help you get and stay sober.

Use Substitutes

Breaking the habit of drinking is made easier by the use of substitutes. The shock of an abrupt change in daily routines is hard to deal with, and this adds to the physical and mental difficulties of the removal of the substance to which one was addicted. However, there are many substitutes that can ease the recovery process that should be considered.

Alcohol is a sugar, and thus sweets can reduce the discomfort of withdrawal and ease recovery. I used chocolate chip cookies when I gave up drinking, and I imposed no limits on cookie-consumption while getting sober. Sweets can provide a nice treat and help reduce the desire to drink. Whatever harm sweets might do in the short term is inconsequential compared to the damage of heavy drinking. Don't even worry about it. All that matters is that you don't drink today, by whatever means necessary.

Don't forget that the main reason we drink is because we are thirsty. Drinking a lot of water will prevent thirst and thus reduce the desire to drink alcohol – especially beer. I was a beer drinker and I found LaCroix (seltzer water in a 12oz can) to be a wonderful substitute. Again, no limits are necessary, drink all the bubbly water you want. This puts a cold carbonated beverage in your hand and allows you to go through the physical motions of drinking. This certainly has a positive effect, reducing the discomfort and social awkwardness of quitting. It also puts other drinkers at ease, as they are going to feel awkward too, seeing their old drinking buddy sitting still without a beer. The substitute helps them too, so drink up the seltzer water, or fruit juice, or mix the two to make a pleasant cocktail. I do not recommend sugary sodas, as they can be very unhealthy. Try to keep your substitutes as healthy as you can, and don't introduce a new problem into your life.

In addition to physical substitutes like cookies and seltzer water, mental substitutes also help us stay sober. Alcohol and drinking trick the drinker into thinking that they are doing something. For example, consider the following dialogue.

Question: "Hey man, whatcha doin?"

Answer: "Drinking beer out on the porch" or "Enjoying a glass of wine" or "Having a sundowner".

These responses all have the guise of activity, as if the drinking were an acceptable pass-time in itself. Alcohol fools us into thinking that we are doing something (television does this too). The reality is that we are doing nothing but slowly poisoning ourselves.

However, the newly-sober will feel anxiety over this new feeling of "doing nothing". The power of addiction is such that our bodies want the alcohol back in our lives (until much time has passed) and will make us feel like we are not doing anything when we are not drinking. Action is needed to overcome this. Exercise and mental challenge fit the bill. Now is a good time to start going to the gym, running, swimming, riding a bicycle, walking, kayaking, sailing, or whatever form of exercise you choose. Now is also a good time to start reading a new book, studying something intensely, picking up an instrument, or learning whatever you want. I became obsessed with sailing while I was getting sober, and read many books about it before finally buying a sailboat.

The truth is that we were not doing anything constructive while we were drinking and now we have the time, energy, and mental capacity to accomplish great things. When we quit drinking and/or taking other drugs, opportunities present themselves. Our minds turn on and become more powerful. We have the ability to exercise and participate in fun sports. We can now organize adventures that were impossible before we got sober. Work will become more efficient. Virtually all aspects of our life will improve with sobriety.

Keep Count of Your Days, Months or Years Sober

Keep an accurate count of the days you have been sober. Each new day is a victory and adds to your count. Keep trying to add one more day to your count. Eventually you will lose count of your days sober, at which time you will be counting months. Each new month is like a birthday, only more significant. Each new year is absolutely huge and worthy of a celebration and a big reward.

Keeping track of our progress strengthens our resolve to stay sober. Celebrating our successes reminds us that we can and will remain sober. Sharing our anniversaries with family, friends, and on social media reminds us of our commitment and our success, and also serves to show others that it can be done.

Count each day sober. Day one is the beginning and represents a great decision on your part. Day two proves that the journey to a new life has begun. Day three is another mountain crossed on our way. Each day is a success and should be regarded as such.

After your first week has passed sober, congratulate yourself. When a month is passed, treat it like a birthday with a real celebration or a gift to yourself, after all, you've saved a lot of money by now. Treat each passing month this way for the foreseeable future. If you quit drinking on the third day of February, like I did, then the third of each month will be like a birthday to you. Whatever the date, remember and cherish it. We need tangible rewards and reminders in order to stay sober.

Your yearly anniversaries are worthy of celebration; they are like birthdays, only more significant. Treat them as such. Celebrate however you feel appropriate, whether it be a gift to yourself, a vacation, or some other treat. It is a big deal to remain sober for a year. Reflect on this, and cherish your new life.

Get Counselling if Necessary

Look into getting counselling. A counsellor is another person to whom we will be accountable, thus increasing our chances for success.

Talking through our issues that led us to our drinking problem is likely necessary and will help our lives in other ways. A good therapist can help us to identify the issues in our lives that may have caused or contributed to our abuse of alcohol (or other drugs). These issues need to be resolved.

Having regular scheduled appointments will serve to remind us of our commitment to staying sober and strengthen our resolve to do so. One common stumbling block to getting and staying sober is the attitude that this was all a silly idea and can just be ignored. This is less likely to occur when we have appointments with a counsellor on our calendar. These appointments will remind us that this is a real problem that we are solving.

An addiction therapist can be a real asset, but beware of anyone who wants to prescribe drugs. I'm no expert on drugs, but drugs are what got us here in the first place, so adding more addictive drugs to our lives is risky. I recommend trying to stay sober without the use of more drugs, especially narcotics.

Medical insurance sometimes covers counselling, so check into this.

Have Someone Check Your Progress Daily

Consider calling a relative and telling them you quit drinking. Ask them to help you stay sober by texting or calling regularly and asking if you are still sober. However, you might need to ask a few people because some will not feel comfortable doing this, or they will forget, or they won't take you seriously.

Telling others we quit has many benefits. There is no longer any need in our society to remain anonymous about alcoholism. The more we come out of the closet and tell people about our struggles, the greater the chance we have to succeed. Being open about addiction also has the positive effect on society of letting other alcoholics know that they are not alone and that sobriety is a possibility.

Our society does so many things wrong and when it seems that everyone is doing something, it appears to be acceptable behavior. Thus, we are all confronted with bad examples to follow. When you find a better path, share it with the world. Lead by example, and let others help you achieve your goals.

Tell Everyone

Don't hide any longer, come out of the closet and tell the world that you have quit drinking. We are all scared of doing this. One reason we are scared is because we are afraid that we will look foolish if we fail. This is the point! When we tell people that we have quit drinking, we become accountable to them. We know that if we fail we will let them down. We will look like a failure. We don't want this, so the accountability therefore increases our chances of success. We are looking for any and all mental tricks that will help us to succeed. The mind is a tricky piece of equipment, and we can indeed use tricks on ourselves to achieve goals. Look for your own tricks and use them.

Share your milestones with friends, loved ones and your social-media network. There is no need to remain anonymous. Your true friends will offer congratulations and support. Doing this also makes you accountable and reduces the chances of a relapse. Remember that anyone who discourages you from remaining sober is either ignorant or in denial of their own alcoholism (or other drug addiction). The younger you and your friends are, the more likely you are to encounter this negativity. Age brings experience and wisdom. Discouragement should be avoided, at least in the beginning of your sobriety, but do not let fear of discouragement prevent you from being frank and open about your sobriety and/or alcoholism.

Telling others on social media is a great way to get the word out. I've found nothing but huge outpourings of support from my friends on social media (Facebook). My posts have also attracted people who want to quit, but aren't sure how. I do all I can to help them get started, avoid relapses, and deal with challenging situations. Mostly though, I simply message them daily with the phrase "still sober?" You can do this too, and you should ask someone to do it for you. We need to be accountable to someone, and we need to be able to share our daily victories with someone.

When other alcoholics see that someone has successfully quit drinking, it encourages them to do the same. It is much easier to continue on the path of alcohol abuse when it seems like everyone else is doing it too. But when we see others, especially friends, getting sober, it makes us reflect on our own drinking habits. Getting sober and sharing our experiences doing so lets others know that it is possible.

There is little need in our society to remain anonymous about our drinking problems. Rather it helps everyone when we are open and frank about alcohol abuse and getting sober.

Do Things You Couldn't Do Before You Got Sober

An important part of our therapy that helps us stay sober is to do things that we couldn't do as a drunk. These activities reward us for sobriety and remind us why we quit drinking. They reinforce our resolve to stay sober.

For example, when I was getting sober I started running, lifting weights, hitting a punching bag, and swimming half-miles in the ocean. I needed adrenaline. Alcohol had taken the place of exciting sports and adventure in my life.

As a drinker of nearly 12 beers a day, my activities were limited to things I could do with a large cooler or refrigerator nearby. Backpacking was out, car camping was in. My dreams of sailing long distances were out, because I'd never be able to bring enough beer and keep it cold.

After ten months of sobriety, I came to realize that I needed to go on a big adventure, one that I couldn't have done sober, so I organized a 5-day canoe trip in the Okefenokee National Wildlife Reserve, a 650 square-mile swamp in southern Georgia. There would have been no way to do this trip before I quit drinking, as I could not have fit all the beer I would have needed in my canoe. I would have had to tow a second canoe behind me packed with coolers.

The trip was a success and a great reward for my efforts at staying sober. It was also a reminder of the limitations that drinking had put on me, and the freedom that I now had.

While in the canoe, I realized how much I liked being surrounded by raw nature, being nomadic, and travelling by boat. I remembered how much I liked sailing.

I then decided to save some of the money that I wasn't spending on beer and use it for a big adventure to celebrate my one year of sobriety anniversary. This line of thinking led me to take a one-week sailing class, which was soon followed by a three-week sailing trip in the Caribbean.

It was during this trip that I was able to quit smoking marijuana. In the beginning of my sobriety, smoking pot helped me to not drink. But as time passed, I realized that it was but another unnecessary addiction that I needed to quit. The vacation facilitated this. Getting out of town, away from my old habits and haunts, away from the temptations, away from the known sources of the weed, helped my situation. I was in a new and interesting environment. I was somewhere where I wasn't constantly reminded of my addiction. I was away from my life and my habits, away from my desk with its drawer containing my smoking paraphernalia, away from my dealers, away from my smoking friends, away from the places in which I smoked and the situations that preempted smoking. Getting away helps, after all, it's a new life we are trying to create for ourselves, and new habits need to be made - old habits deleted.

There are probably things that you would like to do, but that alcohol prevented you from doing. Think deeply about this and come up with a list. Each one of these things accomplished will strengthen your resolve to stay sober. Each one is a tangible reward for having given up drinking. Each one will enrich your life and serve as a reminder that life while sober is better than life while drunk and hungover. We need to remind ourselves of this, because the devil that is alcoholism will be pushing the opposite sentiment, and we need to overpower the devil. Get out into the world and experience it, alcoholism tends to make us want to spend our time at bars, or in front of the TV, doing things that do not enrich our lives, but rather make us sick and broke the next day. Sobriety allows us to enjoy sunrises, great adventures, financial success, good health, mental growth, and much more.

Use the Money You Have Saved for a Reward

Our brains respond to rewards and the promise of rewards. Nearly everything we are motivated to do has a reward at the end. The promise of a reward increases motivation, and we need to maximize our motivation to stay sober in order to succeed in staying sober. The alcohol used to give us a daily reward, and our brains became very accustomed to this. We need to promise ourselves a reward for staying sober. The promise of good health and happiness in the future is not enough. We need something tangible and fun! Not buying alcohol will save us a lot of money, so decide what reward will work for you. In the beginning, a weekly reward is a good idea, like a dinner out, or a small but fun purchase. Monthly rewards are a big deal, and your completion of a year is huge!

After a year has passed, treat yourself to something really special. Plan how you will celebrate your one-year anniversary well in advance, it's never too soon to start thinking about it. Save money for this throughout your first year, and save cash. Put cash that you would have spent on alcohol in a box and occasionally pull it out and look at it. Count the money and think about how this money would have been wasted on drunkenness and hangovers. Think of the productive things you did instead, and look at the money. Think of how you will spend this money. Maybe you have children and want to spend it on them. Maybe you want to go on the vacation you've been dreaming about. Perhaps your house or car needs repairs that you've been putting off. Or perhaps you have a master plan to re-create your life and the cash will provide a springboard into this new you.

Now put some more cash in the pile and put it all back in the box. Remember this box of money and think about it when you need to strengthen your resolve.

Don't Go Back to Drinking, Ever

This may seem like a contradiction to the concept presented earlier of not thinking about having to stay sober in the future, but it is very important to never go back. After having stayed sober for a while, it's common to begin to think that we can eventually go back and be a responsible drinker. But if you are predisposed to addiction, like maybe ten percent of humans are, then it is impossible to go back to drinking and be like those that are not predisposed to addiction. The devil will awaken within you and the devil will regain control.

We must not go back ever. We must remind ourselves in various ways to not go back to drinking. Helping others get and stay sober is one way to remind ourselves of our commitment. Talking openly about staying sober helps. Whatever we can do to remind ourselves not to start drinking again will help. I named my sailboat Sobrius (Latin for sobriety) for this reason. You will have to come up with your own way to remind yourself of your commitment, and it must be done.

Being open and frank about our sobriety and our past abuse of alcohol is a useful way to remind ourselves of our commitment. It is simply too easy to give up and go back if we are anonymous about our alcoholism. Rather, we should not hide our past, nor should we hide our sober present or our sober future.

Lead by Example

I've found it best not to preach to drinkers; leading by example is quite enough. You can keep your friends who still drink if you do not demand that they quit too. There are exceptions to this, of course, but for the most part it's best not to talk down to those who still drink, nor to chastise them for drinking. They will see you not drinking; they will see you becoming healthier; they will see you losing weight; they will see that you have more money; they will see you achieving new and wonderful goals. This is quite enough. Some of them will follow your lead without you having said a word to them about their habit.

Humans are programmed to imitate. This is how we learn to speak. This is how culture develops. This is how trends form. This is how many of us started drinking in the first place. So instead of hiding your sobriety, be openly sober and others will follow. They will be especially encouraged to follow if they can see our sobriety leading us to new heights, new achievements, and new health.

Being open about my alcoholism and my sobriety on social media has led others to follow my example, and this I consider to be one of the greatest things I have achieved in my life. When I think about the possibility that I have helped others get sober, it gives me a wonderful feeling inside, like I have made the world a better place, increasing my store of karma and making my life better. We can't lead by example if we remain anonymous, so come out of the closet and let the world know how good sobriety has been to you.

Make Your Dreams Come True

Sobriety brings about the ingredients of dreams. With more free time, more mental power, and more money, we can now achieve our dreams. We need to think long and hard about what we really want to accomplish with the rest of our lives. Think about what other great people have done. They were normal people just like us, but they set high goals and worked hard to achieve them. Now it is our time to do just this. Our new sobriety is like a super-power that we can use to reach new heights.

We need to think deeply about what makes us happy and why this makes us happy. Then we need to come up with activities or goals that will lead us to this happiness. Next, we need to formulate a plan to allow us to do what makes us happy. We must determine what the first small step is in this plan. We must do this. Great achievements start with small steps. Take the first small step, then the second. As we accomplish these first steps, the rest of the plan will seem much less intimidating. Finally, we will realize that the plan is going to come to fruition, and we take the final steps and achieve our goals. When you do achieve your goal, remember that sobriety got you there. Remember that alcohol kept this achievement from you. Remember that you do not drink anymore, and that you will never go back to the devil that is alcohol.

Tell Yourself "I Don't Drink Anymore"

This is a phrase that we need to repeat to ourselves. We must create a new identity, and the new identity does not drink alcohol. We are no longer drinkers. We don't drink anymore. Repeating this phrase will help us recreate ourselves. It is another mental trick, like reprogramming our brains. Our brains are like computers, and we can program them through study, repetition, meditation, prayer, and conscious effort. We live inside our minds, so make your mind the kind of place in which you want to live – clean, strong, orderly, a place that encourages success.

Keep the phrase "I don't drink anymore" ready to use, like a tool in the pocket. When a trying situation arises, we can use this tool like a Swiss Army Knife. When we feel a craving coming on, or we encounter a situation that reminds us of our past life as a drinker, we need only repeat the phrase "I don't drink anymore". Say this to yourself as often as you can, as repetition brings about mental change.

Meditation strengthens our ability to control our mind, and since our mind controls our body, meditation also strengthens our ability to control bodily functions. Overcoming alcoholism requires both mental and physical fortitude. Our mind needs to be able to resist the urge to drink, and our body needs to overcome the effects of withdrawal.

Meditation can take many forms, but mainly entails clearing the mind of all thoughts and focusing on the moment, the breath, the scene, or the sounds around us. Let conscious thoughts pass and fade; try to empty the mind of thoughts, like turning off the television. This is an exercise, like lifting weights to strengthen muscles, but instead it strengthens mind.

Remember, you don't drink anymore.

Determine Why You Drank So Much

Look inside yourself and ask the question: "Why did I drink so much?".

There could be an unsolved issue in your psyche that caused the drinking. Perhaps something from your childhood is making you angry. Look back into your childhood and try to determine what you are still upset about. Think deeply about this. Imagine that the adult in you is having a conversation with the child in you, the child that you were in the past, the child that is still upset. Have the adult tell the child to let it go, the past is over, and to move on. The anger is hurting you and needs to be stopped. There is no logic in hurting yourself. Let the anger go, and look to the future instead.

Perhaps there is a fear in you that needs to be overcome. Stepping out of our comfort zone is beneficial. We should all do this and try to get over our fears, especially the irrational ones. Fears can be overcome by facing them. Facing one's fears is easiest done in baby steps. Take in what you are afraid of in small doses, then increase the exposure later. Eventually you will find that you are stronger and braver than you thought. Overcoming our fears should be a life-goal and a high priority. Fears are limiting. They make our worlds smaller and reduce our options and opportunities. As a sober person, your mind will be functioning on a higher level, and fears will fall by the wayside.

Take Note of Improvements Gained Through Sobriety

Sobriety brings about many improvements in our lives, and we need to recognize these and celebrate them in order to appreciate our sobriety. It is easy to forget or to get discouraged when we reach a plateau, so keeping track of improvements and milestones helps us maintain our motivation to stay sober; fully appreciating our sobriety will help us to remain sober long-term.

Take note of your improved health. You have probably lost weight, so step onto a scale regularly. Remember your weight before you quit and compare it to your current weight. If you weigh less now, that is a success worthy of celebration. Every time you weigh yourself, compare your current weight to that before you quit drinking. This should be a continuous reminder of your success over alcohol and your commitment to stay sober.

Alcohol depletes our ability to fight off disease, and thus we get sick more often when we drink. Being sober allows the immune system to function as it should. Chances are you will get sick far less as a sober person. Take note of this. When was the last time you got sick? Are you getting sick less often since you got sober? I don't think I got sick once in my first two years of sobriety, compared to multiple times a year before I quit drinking.

Being healthy allows us to work more and earn more - another payoff from sobriety. Showing up on time for work, being reliable, responsible and more productive will pay off big in the long-run. Sobriety brings financial success. Take note of how much money you make and congratulate yourself if earnings increase while you are sober. Alcohol was holding you down, and now you are climbing out of the hole it had caused you to dig.

Your emotional state, mood, and general happiness should improve with sobriety. Alcohol becomes a tool of the alcoholic to alter our mood. When we are drinking, we eventually come to a state in which we are incapable of being happy unless we are drinking. Our bodies must adapt to the sudden change upon getting sober. The tool we once relied on for happiness is withheld from us. We become depressed and crave happiness, which we used to find in alcohol. But our minds and bodies adapt and we learn how to feel pleasure and happiness without the drug. As time passes we begin to feel happy more often, eventually attaining an emotional state far superior to that which we endured as a drunk.

It is the nature of drug use to make us feel wonderful in the beginning. We experiment with a new drug, and it makes us feel good. We have a fabulous time using the drug and then we want it more and more. It becomes our new friend. But eventually we don't feel right unless we are using the drug. We go from getting high to getting straight. Instead of elevating our mood to something above normal, we come to need the drug simply to feel normal. As we approach the final state of alcoholism or drug addiction, we are absolutely sick until we use the drug, at which point we feel normal, but this normal is way below the normal we were used to before we became addicted. This process happens slowly, like an alligator drifting through the weeds. We do not realize it is happening, but it does happen to us all. The gator drags us to the bottom of the swamp and rolls us through the mud. Many of us do not survive drug addiction. Alcohol kills 2.5 million people a year, accounting for 4% of all deaths globally, according to the World Health Organization. The only way out is abstinence and recovery. We experience withdrawal, and we recover and regain our health and our happiness. We either win or we lose. There is no middle ground for the alcoholic.

As you get sober and your mind starts working as it should, you will likely have problems to solve, problems that were disregarded while drinking. As the alcoholic wakes up from the nightmare of life as a sick and irresponsible drunk, these problems will become visible. They are not new. They are not caused by sobriety. Rather they are made visible by our sobriety. This visibility is a blessing. It is an opportunity to fix our problems and thus improve our lives. See them, note them, make strategies to fix them. You don't need to solve all of your problems today. It might be enough to simply note them as they arise. The solutions will appear too; execute them. As these issues are solved, the life of the recovering alcoholic improves. Our confidence builds, our resolve strengthens, and our goals get achieved. We learn to live again.

Help Others Get and Stay Sober

Helping other problem drinkers get sober has many benefits both to us and to society; it is a crucial part of our therapy. As a general rule, lead by example. Most people don't like to be told what to do and might immediately want to do the opposite of what someone is demanding they do. Do not preach. Do not demand. Do not bring up the subject of other people's drinking (of course there can be exceptions to this). Talk openly and frankly about your own sobriety, but don't offend those who still drink.

People who drink will often feel uncomfortable around those of us who don't. Problem drinkers will be more uncomfortable, as they will be faced with their own alcoholism. Do not judge them, and do not berate them for drinking. It's not necessary and will likely work against you. Instead, lead by example. Show them that sobriety is possible; show them that sobriety is healthy; show them that sobriety brings inner peace and happiness.

If you are open about your sobriety, people will eventually come to you seeking advice or help. This may be subtle, so be ready to recognize when someone is reaching out and wants your help. They may simply ask how you got sober, or how you maintain your sobriety. Share with them all you can, and ask them if they want to get sober.

Tell them that it helps to have someone to whom they are accountable, someone who will ask daily if they are still sober, someone to offer advice when needed.

Tell them that you can be this person for them, and then do it, regardless of their response. You can use your own judgement regarding how often to check up on them, but I've found that at least for the first month, daily contact works, tapering off throughout the first year. Try to remember the date they quit, and congratulate them every month, and on their one-year anniversary.

I simply send the message "still sober?". If they respond that they are in fact still sober, then follow up with a congratulation like "good job!" or "that's awesome! Keep it up!". This allows them to share their success and receive a daily reward for their struggles. This also serves to legitimize their struggle, as you clearly understand just how hard it is to abstain from a substance that is physically-addictive and a habit that is ingrained and part of their self-image. Let them know you understand. Your daily message also opens the door to conversation, allowing them to ask for specific advice or to vent their troubles. Your responses will not only help them, but they will also help you to organize your thoughts and consider your own strategies for staying sober.

If, however, their response is negative and they are drinking again, your goal is to real them back in, like a fish, but unfortunately it is alcohol that has the hook and the line, while you are armed only with logic and psychology.

Do not judge; do not berate, but put yourself in their position. Ask yourself what would work for you – what words would get you to put down the drink and try again to get sober? Be understanding, but firm. If they responded at all, it's because they want to maintain contact with you – their lifeline to sobriety. They'd rather be sober, or else they would not have responded at all.

Tell your friend who has relapsed something like "It's alright, this happens, let's try again. Tomorrow will be day one. Don't give up, you can do this." Don't give up on them. Helping someone get sober is a huge accomplishment and sometimes takes a lot of effort.

If someone you have been contacting does not respond at all, give them some time, then try again. If they started drinking again, and they have not responded to your "still sober?" message, then they don't want to hear from you right now. Give them some space, but don't give up on them. Try again in the near-future. On the other hand, they might still be sober and just don't want to respond for some other reason. Use your own judgement, experiment with the timing of the "still sober?" messages, but don't be scared to send them. The system works, and you will feel good about yourself when you see the results.

There really is nothing like helping someone get sober. When you do so, you are making the world a better place, and it's not just one person you are helping. You are helping everyone they interact with, their family, co-workers, friends, etc… Sobriety spreads - other people see them get sober, and they directly help others get sober. When you help one person get sober, you might be helping a hundred people get sober.

Most of the people that have come to me for help did so through Facebook after reading my posts about my journey to sobriety. They contacted me via messenger with a question about my sobriety and thus the dialogue started.

The following is a transcript of messages from a woman who was a friend of a friend. She saw my Facebook posts about getting sober and started the following conversation via Facebook messenger:

July 29, 2016

Her: I see your success when my friend likes them. I pay attention. A glimpse of what's possible. I continue on with my years of struggle… a serious struggle… Sick of going back for more. How do you do it?

Me: Do you want to quit drinking?

Her: Yes. Totally.

Me: Have you had a drink today?

Her: No

Me: Good. Let's try not to drink today. When you feel a craving, recognize it as a symptom of your condition, which you will overcome. Each time you reject this craving recognize this as a victory. Instead of drinking tonight do something productive. Message me in the morning to tell me that you were successful and we will take it from there. Stay in touch today if you need more support, and let me know in the evening how you are doing.

Her: OK. I'll do it. I will do it. Thank you for your help.

Me: Great! If you have any alcohol in the house I recommend pouring it out, down the toilet (where it belongs) and taking a picture of the act. This photo will serve as a reminder of your commitment. If you do this, send me a picture. If you are not ready for this step, skip it. But stay sober today.

Her: I don't have any in the house. My MO is to buy it after work and drink it all night. Sometimes I resist stopping only to blindly get into my car that evening and drive to one of the four liquor stores near my house. I didn't have a drop on Wednesday, but I did yesterday. I'm not drinking today.

Me: I was the same way. I bought a 12-pack every day. Just think about tonight and stay sober. You'll wake up without a hangover tomorrow. Today is day one. Count the days you stay sober. Each one is a terrific victory.

Her: Thank you so much. I feel pretty positive right now. I didn't make a pit stop.

Me: That's a victory! Keep them coming.

Her: Right on. Victory and freedom.

Me: That's right!

Me: Substitutes are helpful. LaCroix and chocolate chip cookies helped me. There's no limit on substitutes when you are getting sober.

July 30

Her: No alcohol yesterday. None. Victory. Woke up w/o a hangover. I'll go get some LaCroix. That's a good idea.

Me: Congratulations!!!
If you can keep it up, the 29th of each month will be like a birthday to you. July 29th is the day your new life started.

Me: However, don't dwell on the future. The only thing that matters is that you don't drink today.

Her: Okay. Just today, Saturday. Thanks again.

That night

Me: Staying sober?

Her: So far… No alcohol. I'm settling in for the night. No drinking. Thanks for checking.

Me: Good job, you are doing it!

Her: Thanks! I've had some thoughts but chose to do other activities.

Me: That's good. The cravings will eventually go away and you will be free.

Her: Good to know that. Encouraging words. Victory and freedom.

Me: They will both be yours soon.

Her: Thank you!

July 31

Her: Whelp, did it. No Alcohol. Difficulty sleeping though. Allowed for some reflective thoughts... like how the F am I still alive after all my reckless drinking. Seriously? How am I not dead? I'm going to stay sober today.

Me: I think I have a guardian angel, or I'd be dead or in jail for DUI. Sleeping should get better than ever soon. It did for me anyway. Stay sober today and do something awesome that you couldn't or wouldn't have done as a drunk.

Her: OK, I'll do both.

Later

Me: still sober?

Her: Yes! Thanks!
Drinking LaCroix right now. This morning I called my mom while sober (I haven't done that in a very long time) and I went to this festival that I haven't been able to go to for the past four years because of being hungover, seriously. One day at a time. No trips to the liquor store today.

Me: That's all great news! Doing things that require sobriety will help you stay sober and enjoy life to its fullest. Good job! Keep it up!

Aug 1

Her: Sober Day 3. Feels like 30. I'm doing it but this is a crazy battle. I took a screen shot of the first thing you said: "good, let's try not to drink today…" I just keep referring to that when I start thinking about drinking. I'm not going to pick up a bottle today.

Me: thumbs up emoji (TU)
Stay sober today!

Her: Thanks! With all my power!

Me: Don't stop at the liquor store!

Her: Didn't and I'm not going to later this afternoon. Thanks again.

Me: I forgot you live two time zones away.

Her: No worries. It really really helps (not sure how but that's OK but it does). Plus, specifically saying I'm not going to drink seems to help me too.

Me: Yes to both. It helps to be accountable to someone, and to share your daily success with them. It is also necessary to frequently remind yourself that you don't drink anymore (or at least not today). Keep up the work, I know it's hard but it gets easy and the rewards are fantastic. Everything in your life will improve.

Her: OK. Got it.

Aug 2

Her: I'm going on my 5th day sober! I thought it was the 4th. Ha! The longest this year since last spring when I stopped for ten days. Thank you for taking the time to help me stay accountable. Thank you. No drinking today = victory and freedom.

Me: Victory five days straight!
I enjoy helping others get sober. You'll probably be doing the same a year from now. It takes someone who's done it to help another do it.

Later
Me: Still sober?

Her: Yes!! Drove right past all the shit. I want this so very, very much.

Me: You are doing it! It only gets easier. Keep your guard up. Is tomorrow one week?

Her: Thursday will be 7 days. I will be totally guarded. I just continue to remind myself that my new life has started. My energy is returning. I'm less irritable. I feel clearer. This day is a victory.

Me: YES! It's a new life. A better life.

Her: Yes. So very much so. Thank you, again.

Aug 3

Me: Still sober?

Her: Yep!!! I feel amazing!

Me: Yay!! :)

Her: I am not drinking today, but I feel like tomorrow will be harder for me. I probably need to just think about today and not tomorrow.

Me: Just don't drink right now. Thinking about not drinking in the future is a classic stumbling block. Cross that bridge...

Some days are harder than others, but once you get sober, you are stronger.

Her: Okay. Get over the bridge. Yes, I'll be stronger. Got it.

Me: You will feel like you have super-powers if you stick it out.

Her: I want that. I'm MORE determined.

Aug 4

Me: Still sober?

Her: Yes. Many aggravating challenges today, but I'm digging deep.

Me: Excellent! I'm very proud of you. Keep working and don't drink right now. Or right now…

Her: Thanks! I will not drink today. I'm working toward that cape.

Me: Wonder Woman is coming soon!

Her: Snap.

Aug 5

Me: Day 8, still sober?

Her: YES!!!!!!!! Yes I am!

Me: TU

Her: My friend's last night in town, they invited me to dinner. I'm not going to order any alcohol today. Zilch. JS

Me: Yes. Good friends don't require you to drink. Will power yields super power!

Her: That's an awesome point! And, I'm holding onto that quote.

Me: Make it yours.

Her: Thank you so very much.

Me: My pleasure. Someday soon you'll be doing the same for others. It's part of our therapy.

Her: Something for me to aspire to. Today I feel hopeful about my life. I feel genuine hope and determination. I have not felt this in a very, very long time.

Me: TU

Aug 6

Her: S.O.B.E.R. Yes!!

Me: Good job, day 9!

Aug 7

Me: Day ten!

Her: I can't believe it. I really can't. I can't help but weep thinking about it. Thank you so much. I'm not going to let my guard down.

Me: TU

Me: I'm proud of you! The first ten days are a HUGE accomplishment. Have you come out of the closet yet and announced your sobriety? I got a ton of support on Facebook.

Her: No. I've been thinking about that though.

Me: It makes it more real.

Her.   I see the support you get… It's overwhelming to me. Bottom line… I'm afraid.

Me: You'll be much more accountable if everyone knows, and thus have more chance for success.

Her: You're right. What if I screw up?

Me: They'll hardly notice. Most people screw up.

Her: Bottom line… I can not screw up. I cannot. I know my life depends on it. I Know it.

Me: Mine too.

Me: Can I connect you on Facebook with another woman who is getting sober? Supporting others is part of our therapy.

Her: Yes

Me: Cool. _____ _____, check my friends

Her: Okay

Me: Still sober?

Her: I'm still sober. 12… I'm thinking about drinking less. Yesterday I posted about my alcoholism and I wanted a drink immediately. I felt an insane amount of anxiety, but I just let it ride out. I feel great now.

Me: That's the right attitude. I'm proud of you! If you succeed then I succeed. Did you get support from your post?

Her: TU

Me: Congrats on coming out on Facebook.

Her: A weight has lifted.

Aug 11

Me: Still sober?

Her: Yep! Approaching level badass.

Me: You are!

Her: But if you could tell me not to drink, that'd be awesome.

Me: Don't drink tonight. You are a success for me, it would hurt me if you drank again. But I wouldn't abandon you. Just don't do it.

Her: Okay, I'm going to stay sober today. Thank you for that.

Me: Do it! Cravings and suffering are symptoms of our condition. Sobriety brings freedom from craving. Sobriety is freedom. Redirect your attention and energy to something positive. Exercise and adventure help.

Her: Got it. I understand. Just returned from the gym. I'm going to slug a punching bag.

Me: Perfect. I bet you are getting healthier and losing any extra weight you might have had.

Her: Yes, all those things are happening. I'm getting my stamina back.

Aug 12

Me: Still sober?

Her: Yep! Yesterday made me stronger today.

Me: Yes! That's how it always works. The more you stay sober, the stronger you get, the easier it gets to stay sober. Good job!

Her: I feel great. Thanks for believing in me!!

Me: You bet! I love doing this. It helps me too. We are accountable to each other. You will be helping others quit soon too. It's part of our therapy.

Her: Tomorrow will be 16 days for me. 16! Last year I stayed sober for 15 days. This is the longest I've been sober since I can remember.

Me: You are winning

Me: I could never go for one day for ten years before I quit (except for once when I was really sick and I was on antibiotics. I'm proud of you. You are joining an elite club of strong people who have overcome the devil.

Her: I'm glad you're here. You've smashed the odds. Bottom line… inspiring

Me: TU

Aug 13

Me: Day 16 is here, congratulations!

Her: Yes!!!! Thank you!!!!!! I have regretted not one single moment in 16 days. Not one. No longer an endless wrestling match with myself. I am not drinking alcohol today. My choice makes me extremely happy.

Me: So is it getting easier?

Her: It seems to be. I'm getting better at getting out of flight mode when I become overwhelmed.

Me: That sounds good, like you are regaining full control.

Her: Yeah, I'm doing my best to get there. I know I can do it.

Me: You can and you will.

Her: TU

Aug 14

Me: Did you get through the weekend sober?

Her: Yep! I sure did!

Me: Excellent! I hope temptation is decreasing.

Her: Totally. I got out of town, but was still reminded of my old habits... Like stopping to get alcohol in small mining towns before backpacking. I skipped them all this time.

Me: Good work. How was backpacking sober?

Her: A-effing-mazing. Seriously. Incredible. I was even able to get up at 2:30 in the a.m. to shoot some stars (lightning bolt emoji)

Me: That sounds like more fun than getting drunk and waking up hungover!

Her: Who would have thought?! Totally was.

Me: TU

Aug 17

Her: Got another sweet day under my belt. This is cool, I realized that I no longer have chronic pain in my conoid ligament since I quit booze. I injured it in 2010, if I'd sleep on it wrong, do plank for too long, or do a handful of push-ups pain would seriously kick in. Seriously. Read some cool articles on how alcohol affects ligaments. I guess I'm finally allowing my body to heal and hydrate. (lightning bolt and rainbow emojis)

Although my friend relapsed once, she is still sober today and living a new and vastly-improved life.

Now that you have read my treatise on sobriety, take the next step and get sober. Stay sober. Your new life awaits!

About the Author

Paul Trammell was born in Dallas Texas on October 10, 1970 to Dr. Willis and Betsy Trammell. Paul has an older brother, Sam, and a younger sister, Elizabeth. The family moved soon after to an Indian Reservation in North Dakota, where his father practiced medicine. Next they moved to New Orleans, and then to his parents' home town of Alexandria Louisiana. As a child, Paul spent all of his free time in the woods, exploring the forest, a bayou, and the farm they lived on in Alexandria. When he was 8 they moved to Charleston West Virginia, where he stayed through high-school. Here Paul had many wonderful adventures in nature: hiking, canoeing, mountain-biking, skiing, spelunking, fishing... However, his adventurous spirit led him to trouble with the law. At 13 years-old he was arrested for shoplifting, at 15 he was arrested for marijuana possession, at 17 he was arrested buying alcohol with a fake ID, and at 19 he was charged with DUI and had to serve a 24-hour jail sentence.

After graduating from high school in 1988, Paul studied Biology at Florida Institute of Technology (FIT) in Melbourne, FL. Here he learned how to surf, which became an obsession. Paul also did a lot of SCUBA diving while in college, both in Florida and The Bahamas. After graduating with a BS in Biology in 1992, Paul continued his studies at West Virginia University (WVU) and in 1995 received an MS in Biology. While at WVU he spent a lot of time mountain-biking, both racing and exploring. After this he taught 9th grade Biology and Algebra at The Cheshire Academy in Cheshire CT. But after one year he moved, disillusioned with teaching, back to WV and got work as a roofer. Soon after he moved to St Augustine, FL where he found work as a frame carpenter, but also chased his dreams by playing guitar in original bands, painting in oils, writing, surfing, and adventuring. He has travelled to surf many times to Costa Rica, and also to Mexico, El Salvador, Chile, and even Ireland. In St Augustine Paul has worked as a realtor, real-estate investor/landlord, bicycle mechanic, Environmental Consultant, and is currently a finish-carpenter. He also plays electric guitar and writes music with his band I-Vibes. His current obsession is offshore sailing, and he lives on his sailboat Sobrius in Jacksonville Florida and has a home in St. Augustine Florida. Keep an eye out for his next book, which will be about sailing on Sobrius.

Acknowledgements

Thanks to my parents for putting up with me when I was a rebellious child, picking me up at the police station four times, and for all their support throughout my life. Thanks to my parents and Dr. Christopher Todd Ruhland for their help editing this book. Thanks to my brother Sam for regularly checking to see if I was still sober in the beginning of my sobriety. Thanks to Missy Yeager for being frank about my alcohol and marijuana problems and bringing them to my attention. Thanks to my sister Elizabeth and her husband Justin Ruby for their support. Thanks to Noah Baxter for helping me realize I had a drinking problem by setting a six-beer daily maximum for me, to which I could not stick. Thanks to Jonti Hays for counselling in the beginning of my effort to get sober. Thanks to Jim Hays for telling me about his sobriety, which sparked interest in me to get sober. Thanks to Cristina Vidal for being frank about my alcohol and marijuana problems and bringing them to my attention. Thanks to my band I-Vibes for supporting me through my struggle getting sober. Thanks to Amazon for supplying me with a format for publishing this book.

Made in the USA
Columbia, SC
01 September 2018